SAFE CAT FOOD RECIPES COOKBOOK

Simple delicious and Easy Homemade meals for your kitty

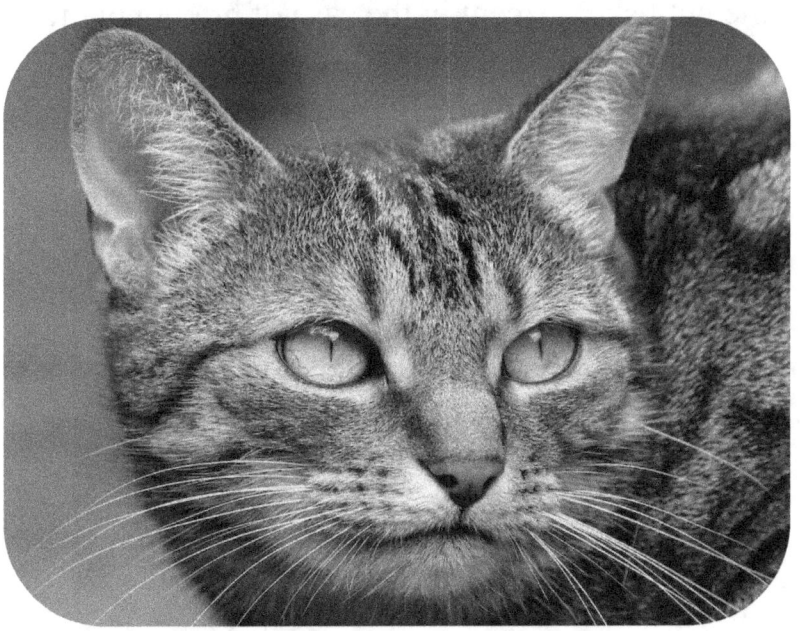

Donald Moon Smith

This book is a work of nonfiction. The views and opinions expressed in this book are solely those of the author and do not necessarily reflect the official policy or position of any organization mentioned. The author and publisher have made every effort to ensure the accuracy of the information herein, but errors and omissions may occur. Readers should consult with a professional where appropriate

TABLE OF CONTENTS

INTRODUCTION 5

Why Homemade Cat Food? 5

Understanding Your Cat's Nutritional Needs 7

CHAPTER 1 8

BASICS OF CAT NUTRITION 8

Essential Nutrients for Cats 8

Understanding Portion Control 10

PRACTICAL TIPS FOR PORTION CONTROL 11

Common Cat Food Allergens 12

CHAPTER 2 13

SAFE INGREDIENTS FOR HOMEMADE CAT FOOD 13

Protein Sources 13

Carbohydrates for Cats 14

Healthy Fats for Feline Friends 14

Vitamins and Minerals 15

CHAPTER 3 16

TOOLS AND EQUIPMENT 16

Choosing the Right Kitchen Tools 16

Safe Food Preparation Practices 18

CHAPTER 4 20

HOMEMADE CAT FOOD RECIPES 20

Beginner's Recipes 20

Simple Chicken and Rice Delight 22

Turkey and Sweet Potato Surprise 24

Intermediate Recipes 26

Tuna and Quinoa Medley 28

Salmon and Pumpkin Feast 30

Advanced Recipe 32

Beef and Liver Gourmet 33

Homemade Fish and Vegetable Blend 35

CHAPTER 5 37

SPECIAL DIETS AND HEALTH CONSIDERATIONS 37

Recipes for Cats with Allergies 37

Senior Cat Diet Plans 39

Homemade Food for Cats with Medical Conditions 41

CHAPTER 6 43

Tips for Feeding Homemade Cat Food 43

Transitioning Your Cat to Homemade Food 43

Monitoring Your Cat's Health 45

Troubleshooting Common Issues 47

CHAPTER 7 50

FREQUENTLY ASKED QUESTIONS 50

How Much Homemade Food Should I Feed My Cat? 50

Can I Use Raw Ingredients in Cat Food? 52

What Supplements are Necessary for Homemade Cat Food?54

Appendix: Resources and References 56

Online Resources for Cat Nutrition 56

CONCLUSION 57

INTRODUCTION

Why Homemade Cat Food?

There are several reasons why some cat owners choose to feed their cats homemade food rather than commercial cat food. Here are some comprehensive reasons for opting for homemade cat food:

Control over Ingredients:

Homemade cat food allows cat owners to have full control over the quality and source of ingredients. This is especially important for cats with allergies or sensitivities to certain ingredients commonly found in commercial cat food.

Tailored Nutrition:

Every cat is unique, and their nutritional needs can vary. Homemade cat food recipes can be tailored to meet the specific dietary requirements of an individual cat, considering factors such as age, weight, health condition, and activity level.

Avoiding Additives and Preservatives:

Commercial cat foods often contain additives, preservatives, and artificial flavors. Homemade cat food recipes enable owners to eliminate these potentially harmful additives, providing a more natural and wholesome diet.

Reducing Fillers:

Some commercial cat foods contain a significant amount of fillers, such as grains and carbohydrates, which may not align with a cat's natural diet. Homemade cat food allows for a higher proportion of animal-based proteins and fats, mimicking a cat's natural carnivorous diet more closely.

Freshness and Flavor: Homemade cat food is prepared in small batches, ensuring freshness and optimal taste. Cats can be picky eaters, and the palatability of homemade food may encourage better eating habits, especially for cats that are reluctant to eat commercial diets.

Minimizing Processed Ingredients:

Commercial cat foods often go through extensive processing, which can reduce the nutritional value of the ingredients. Homemade cat food recipes involve minimal processing, preserving the nutrient content of the ingredients.

Addressing Medical Conditions:

Cats with specific medical conditions, such as diabetes, kidney disease, or food allergies, may benefit from a customized homemade diet that caters to their unique health needs. A veterinarian's guidance is crucial in formulating recipes for cats with medical issues.

Building a Bond:

The act of preparing homemade cat food can strengthen the bond between the cat owner and their feline companion. It involves hands-on care and attention to the cat's well-being, fostering a deeper connection.

Quality Assurance: Homemade cat food provides a level of transparency and assurance regarding the quality of ingredients used. Owners can choose high-quality, ethically sourced ingredients, promoting the overall health and well-being of their cats.

Understanding Your Cat's Nutritional Needs

Understanding your cat's nutritional needs is paramount to ensuring its overall health and well-being. Cats are obligate carnivores, meaning they thrive on a diet primarily consisting of animal-based proteins. Unlike omnivores, they have specific dietary requirements that include essential amino acids, taurine, arachidonic acid, and various vitamins and minerals that are found in animal tissues.

Proteins are crucial for muscle development, energy, and maintaining a healthy coat, making them a cornerstone of a cat's diet. Taurine, an amino acid found predominantly in animal tissues, is essential for heart health and overall feline vitality. Additionally, arachidonic acid, a type of omega-6 fatty acid, is vital for maintaining healthy skin, coat, and reproductive function.

Understanding portion control is equally important. Cats may not regulate their food intake as effectively as dogs, making it essential to provide appropriately sized servings. Overfeeding can lead to obesity and related health issues, while underfeeding can result in malnutrition.

Considering these factors, cat owners must choose nutritionally balanced diets or formulate homemade recipes under the guidance of a veterinarian. Regular veterinary check-ups and a keen awareness of feline dietary preferences ensure that a cat receives the nutrients it needs for a vibrant and healthy life.

CHAPTER 1

BASICS OF CAT NUTRITION

Essential Nutrients for Cats

Ensuring your feline companion receives the right balance of essential nutrients is crucial for its overall health and longevity. Cats have unique dietary needs as obligate carnivores, requiring specific nutrients that are predominantly found in animal-based sources. Here are key essential nutrients for cats:

Protein: Essential for muscle development, energy, and maintaining a healthy coat, protein is a fundamental component of a cat's diet. Quality protein sources include meat, poultry, and fish.

Taurine: A critical amino acid for cats, taurine is essential for heart health, vision, and reproductive function. Cats cannot synthesize enough taurine on their own, so it must be obtained through their diet, primarily from animal tissues like heart and liver.

Arachidonic Acid: An omega-6 fatty acid, arachidonic acid is vital for maintaining healthy skin, coat, and reproductive function in cats. It is abundant in animal fats and oils.

Vitamins: Cats require various vitamins, including vitamin A for vision, vitamin D for calcium absorption, and vitamin E for immune function. These can be found in balanced amounts in animal-based diets.

Minerals: Essential minerals such as calcium, phosphorus, magnesium, and potassium are crucial for bone health, enzyme function, and overall metabolic processes. These minerals are naturally present in meat and bones.

Fatty Acids: Omega-3 and omega-6 fatty acids, derived from fish oil and animal fats, are essential for maintaining healthy skin, a glossy coat, and supporting immune function.

Examples of nutrient-rich cat-friendly foods include:

Chicken Liver: Rich in protein, taurine, and other essential nutrients.

Salmon: Provides omega-3 fatty acids and high-quality protein.

Beef: A good source of iron and zinc.

Egg Yolks: Contain taurine and various vitamins.

It is important to balance these nutrients in a cat's diet promotes optimal health. All the same, it's essential to consult with a veterinarian to tailor the diet to your cat's specific needs and ensure it meets all nutritional requirements.

Understanding Portion Control

Understanding portion control is a fundamental aspect of maintaining a cat's health and preventing issues like obesity or malnutrition. Unlike some animals, cats may not naturally regulate their food intake, relying on their owners to provide appropriate portions. Here's why understanding portion control is crucial for feline well-being:

Preventing Obesity: Cats are susceptible to obesity, which can lead to various health problems, including diabetes, arthritis, and cardiovascular issues. Controlling portion sizes helps manage calorie intake, preventing excess weight gain.

Meeting Nutritional Needs: Proper portion control ensures that a cat receives the right balance of essential nutrients. Each component of their diet, from proteins to fats and carbohydrates, needs to be provided in the correct amounts to meet their specific dietary requirements.

Individual Variability: Cats have unique nutritional needs based on factors such as age, weight, activity level, and health status. Portion control allows owners to adjust the quantity of food to suit their cat's individual needs, promoting overall well-being.

Avoiding Underfeeding: Inadequate portion sizes can lead to malnutrition and deficiencies in essential nutrients. Understanding a cat's specific dietary requirements helps prevent underfeeding, ensuring they receive the necessary nourishment for optimal health.

Monitoring Changes: Portion control facilitates the monitoring of a cat's eating habits and sudden changes in appetite or weight can be indicative of underlying health.

PRACTICAL TIPS FOR PORTION CONTROL

Read Feeding Guidelines: Follow the recommended feeding guidelines on cat food packaging, but be flexible based on your cat's unique needs.

Weigh Portions: Use a kitchen scale to measure food accurately, especially if your cat requires precise portion control due to health concerns.

Consult with a Veterinarian: A veterinarian can provide guidance on portion sizes based on your cat's age, weight, and health status.

Monitor Body Condition: Regularly assess your cat's body condition to ensure they maintain a healthy weight.

By understanding and implementing proper portion control, cat owners play a vital role in maintaining their feline companions' health and ensuring they lead long, happy lives.

Common Cat Food Allergens

Awareness of common cat food allergens is crucial for cat owners to ensure the well-being of their feline companions. Allergies in cats can manifest as various symptoms, including itching, gastrointestinal upset, and respiratory issues. Identifying and avoiding common cat food allergens can help alleviate these issues. Here are some of the most prevalent allergens:

Chicken and Beef: While these are staple protein sources in many cat foods, some cats can develop allergies to chicken or beef. Allergies to these meats can lead to skin irritations, digestive problems, or even respiratory issues.

Fish: Fish is a common allergen for cats. Allergic reactions may result in skin problems, vomiting, or diarrhea. Additionally, some cats may be sensitive to specific types of fish, such as tuna or salmon.

Dairy: Contrary to popular belief, many adult cats are lactose intolerant. Feeding them dairy products can lead to gastrointestinal issues, including diarrhea. It's essential to avoid milk and other dairy treats unless specifically formulated for lactose-intolerant cats.

Grains: Grains like wheat, corn, and soy are common fillers in commercial cat foods. However, some cats may develop allergies or sensitivities to these ingredients, resulting in digestive upset, skin problems, or ear infections.

Artificial Additives: Artificial colors, flavors, and preservatives can cause adverse reactions in some cats. Allergic responses may vary but can include gastrointestinal upset, lethargy, or skin issues.

CHAPTER 2

SAFE INGREDIENTS FOR HOMEMADE CAT FOOD

Protein Sources

Protein is a fundamental component of a cat's diet, essential for maintaining muscle mass, promoting a healthy coat, and supporting overall vitality. Choosing the right protein sources is crucial to meet a cat's unique nutritional needs as obligate carnivores. High-quality animal-based proteins are optimal, as they provide essential amino acids that cats cannot produce on their own.

Common protein sources in cat food include:

Chicken: Lean and easily digestible, chicken is a popular protein source in many cat diets.

Turkey: Similar to chicken, turkey is rich in protein and often well-tolerated by cats.

Fish: While a good source of omega-3 fatty acids, some cats may be sensitive to certain types of fish.

Beef: A nutritious red meat option, beef provides essential nutrients like iron and zinc.

Lamb: An alternative protein source that can be suitable for cats with sensitivities to more common meats.

Carbohydrates for Cats

While cats are obligate carnivores with a primary need for animal-based proteins, carbohydrates play a limited role in their natural diet. Cats derive energy mainly from proteins and fats, and excessive carbohydrate consumption can lead to health issues. However, some carbohydrates can be included in cat diets for fiber, energy, and nutrient balance. Carbohydrates like rice, oats, and sweet potatoes are easily digestible and can provide a source of energy. It's essential to focus on complex carbohydrates that release energy gradually, preventing spikes in blood sugar levels. Nevertheless, excessive reliance on carbohydrates, especially in the form of fillers like corn or wheat, can contribute to obesity and other health concerns in cats. When incorporating carbohydrates into a cat's diet, it's crucial to strike a careful balance and consult with a veterinarian to ensure the overall nutritional adequacy of the feline diet.

Healthy Fats for Feline Friends

Healthy fats are essential for a cat's overall well-being, contributing to various physiological functions. Omega-3 and omega-6 fatty acids, in particular, play crucial roles in maintaining a cat's skin and coat health, supporting immune function, and promoting proper growth and development. Fatty acids like DHA and EPA, found in fish oil, are vital for cognitive function and vision in cats.

Quality sources of healthy fats in a cat's diet include fish (such as salmon), poultry, and certain plant oils. These fats not only provide energy but also aid in the absorption of fat-soluble vitamins, ensuring optimal nutrient utilization. Moderation is key, as excessive fat intake can lead to obesity, a common concern in cats.

Vitamins and Minerals

Vitamins and minerals are essential components of a cat's diet, playing vital roles in various physiological processes. These micronutrients are critical for maintaining overall health, supporting growth, and preventing nutritional deficiencies. Cats require specific vitamins, such as vitamin A for vision, vitamin D for calcium absorption, and vitamin E for immune function. Essential minerals like calcium, phosphorus, magnesium, and potassium are crucial for bone health, enzyme function, and maintaining a proper balance of bodily fluids.

When you balance the intake of vitamins and minerals is crucial for a cat's well-being. While commercial cat foods are formulated to meet these nutritional needs, homemade diets should be carefully planned with the guidance of a veterinarian to ensure they are complete and well-rounded. Regular veterinary check-ups help monitor and address any potential nutrient imbalances, ensuring that feline companions receive the necessary micronutrients for optimal health and longevity.

CHAPTER 3

TOOLS AND EQUIPMENT

Choosing the Right Kitchen Tools

Selecting the appropriate kitchen tools is paramount when preparing homemade cat food to ensure efficiency, safety, and the preservation of nutritional quality. Here's a guide to choosing the right kitchen tools for the task:

Cutting Tools: Invest in high-quality knives for precision when portioning meat and vegetables. Sharp knives make the process smoother and safer, minimizing the risk of accidents.

Cutting Boards: Choose non-porous cutting boards made of materials like plastic or glass, which are easy to clean and reduce the likelihood of bacterial contamination. Designate specific boards for meat and vegetables to prevent cross-contamination.

Food Processor or Blender: These tools are essential for finely chopping or pureeing ingredients, especially if your cat prefers smoother textures. Opt for a durable and easy-to-clean appliance.

Cookware: Stainless steel or ceramic pots and pans are ideal for cooking cat food. Avoid non-stick coatings that may release harmful chemicals when exposed to high temperatures.

Measuring Utensils: Accurate measurements are crucial for creating balanced and nutritious cat meals. Invest in measuring cups and spoons to ensure precision in portioning ingredients.

Food Scale: A digital kitchen scale is invaluable for measuring ingredients by weight, offering greater accuracy in portion control, especially for meat.

Storage Containers: Choose airtight containers made of glass or BPA-free plastic to store homemade cat food safely. Proper storage helps maintain freshness and prevents contamination.

Thermometer: Ensure meat is cooked to a safe temperature by using a kitchen thermometer. This is crucial for preventing bacterial contamination and ensuring your cat's safety.

Can Opener: If your recipe includes canned ingredients, a reliable can opener is essential. Opt for a sturdy, easy-to-use model for convenience.

Cleaning Supplies: Keep dish soap, sponges, and other cleaning supplies handy for maintaining a clean and hygienic kitchen environment. Regular cleaning keeps hazardous microorganisms at bay. By selecting the right kitchen tools, cat owners can streamline the process of preparing homemade cat food while ensuring the safety and nutritional quality of the meals. Regular maintenance and cleaning of these tools are equally important to uphold hygiene standards in the kitchen.

Safe Food Preparation Practices

Safe food preparation practices are paramount when creating homemade cat food to ensure the health and well-being of your feline companion. Adhering to proper hygiene standards and employing safe handling techniques mitigates the risk of contamination and the transmission of harmful bacteria. Here's a comprehensive guide to safe food preparation practices:

Hand Hygiene: Wash hands thoroughly with soap and water before and after handling raw ingredients. This reduces the risk of introducing contaminants to the food.

Separation of Ingredients: Use separate cutting boards and utensils for raw meat and other ingredients to prevent cross-contamination. Clean and sanitize tools between uses.

Temperature Control: Keep perishable ingredients refrigerated until use and cook meat to a safe internal temperature. Promptly refrigerate any leftovers.

Thorough Cooking: Ensure that meat and other ingredients are cooked thoroughly to eliminate harmful bacteria. Use a food thermometer to verify internal temperatures.

Avoiding Raw Diets: While some cat owners choose raw diets, it's essential to be aware of the associated risks, including bacterial contamination. If opting for raw food, source high-quality ingredients and follow strict hygiene practices.

Cleaning and Sanitizing: Regularly clean and sanitize kitchen surfaces, utensils, and equipment to prevent the growth of harmful bacteria. This is especially critical when working with fresh meat.

Safe Food Handling: Use safe food handling practices, such as defrosting meat in the refrigerator rather than at room temperature. Additionally, avoid leaving food unattended to prevent spoilage.

Storage Practices: Store cat food in airtight containers in the refrigerator or freezer to maintain freshness and prevent bacterial growth. Label containers with the preparation date for monitoring.

Regular Check-ups: Ensure your cat receives regular veterinary check-ups to monitor its health. Any signs of illness should be promptly addressed, and adjustments to the homemade diet may be necessary under veterinary guidance.

Education and Consultation: Stay informed about safe food preparation practices and consult with a veterinarian to ensure the nutritional adequacy of homemade cat food. Professional guidance helps create a balanced and safe diet tailored to your cat's unique needs.

By adhering to these safe food preparation practices, cat owners can provide their feline companions with nutritious homemade meals while minimizing the risk of foodborne illnesses. It's crucial to prioritize hygiene, proper cooking techniques, and regular veterinary oversight to ensure the well-being of your cat.

CHAPTER 4

HOMEMADE CAT FOOD RECIPES

Beginner's Recipes

For cat owners venturing into the realm of homemade cat food, creating beginner-friendly recipes ensures a smooth transition and helps establish a foundation for a balanced diet. Here are two simple and nutritious recipes suitable for beginners:

1. Simple Chicken and Rice Delight:

Ingredients:

One cup cooked and shredded boneless, skinless chicken breast

1/2 cup of cooked brown rice

1 tablespoon of chicken broth (low-sodium)

1 tablespoon of cooked and pureed vegetables (e.g., carrots or peas)

Optional: a teaspoon of fish oil for added omega-3 fatty acids

Instructions: Cook the chicken fully before shredding it into bite-sized pieces.

In a mixing bowl, combine the shredded chicken, cooked brown rice, pureed vegetables, and chicken broth.

Mix the ingredients well to ensure an even distribution.

Optional: Drizzle fish oil over the mixture for additional nutritional benefits.

Serve in your cat's dish, and adjust portions based on your cat's size and dietary needs.

2. Turkey and Sweet Potato Surprise:

Ingredients:

1/2 cup of ground turkey (cooked)

1/4 cup of mashed sweet potatoes

1 tablespoon of turkey or chicken broth (low-sodium)

1 teaspoon of finely chopped parsley (optional for added flavor)

1/4 teaspoon of taurine supplement (consult your veterinarian for appropriate dosage)

Instructions: Cook the ground turkey thoroughly and set it aside to cool.

In a bowl, combine the cooked turkey, mashed sweet potatoes, chopped parsley, and turkey or chicken broth.

Mix the ingredients well until they form a uniform consistency.

Add a taurine supplement, ensuring it is well-distributed in the mixture.

Serve this delightful turkey and sweet potato blend to your cat, adjusting portions as needed.

Simple Chicken and Rice Delight

The "Simple Chicken and Rice Delight" is a beginner-friendly homemade cat food recipe designed to provide essential nutrients in a palatable and easily digestible form. This recipe strikes a balance between lean protein, complex carbohydrates, and a touch of vegetables, ensuring a wholesome meal for your feline friend.

Ingredients: Boneless, skinless chicken breast: This high-quality protein source contributes to muscle development and overall vitality. Cooking and shredding the chicken make it easy for cats to consume.

Brown rice: A source of complex carbohydrates, brown rice adds fiber to the diet, aiding in digestion and providing a sustained release of energy.

Chicken broth: Low-sodium chicken broth enhances the flavor while maintaining hydration. It also helps achieve the desired consistency for the meal.

Cooked and pureed vegetables: Vegetables like carrots or peas introduce vitamins and minerals to the recipe, contributing to a well-rounded nutritional profile.

Instructions: Cook and shred the chicken: Thoroughly cook the chicken breast and shred it into small, feline-friendly pieces. This ensures the protein is easily digestible and enjoyable for your cat.

Prepare the rice: Cook the brown rice separately. Brown rice is chosen for its nutritional value and digestibility.

Combine ingredients: In a mixing bowl, combine the shredded chicken, cooked brown rice, a tablespoon of chicken broth, and the pureed vegetables. This step ensures a uniform distribution of ingredients, offering a balanced blend.

Optional: Add fish oil: For an extra nutritional boost, a teaspoon of fish oil can be drizzled over the mixture. Fish oil is rich in omega-3 fatty acids, supporting skin health and providing additional benefits.

Serve to your cat: Portion the Simple Chicken and Rice Delight according to your cat's size and dietary needs. Monitor your cat's response to ensure they enjoy and tolerate the new homemade meal.

This recipe is not only nutritious but also serves as an excellent introduction to homemade cat food. However, individual cats may have unique dietary requirements, you may consider consulting with a veterinarian in order to tailor the recipe to your cat's specific needs and ensure it meets all nutritional standards.

Turkey and Sweet Potato Surprise

The "Turkey and Sweet Potato Surprise" is a delectable homemade cat food recipe designed with simplicity and nutrition in mind. Tailored for beginners in the world of homemade cat cuisine, this recipe combines the lean protein of turkey with the nutritional benefits of sweet potatoes, create a supper that's not only delectable but also filled with important nutrients.

Ingredients:

Ground turkey: A high-quality, lean protein source that supports muscle development and overall health in cats.

Mashed sweet potatoes: Rich in vitamins, minerals, and dietary fiber, sweet potatoes contribute to digestive health and provide a natural source of sweetness.

Turkey or chicken broth (low-sodium): Enhances flavor and moisture while maintaining a low sodium content for optimal feline health.

Finely chopped parsley (optional): Add a touch of freshness and flavor, making the meal even more appealing to cats.

Taurine supplement (optional): Taurine is an essential amino acid for cats, and a supplement can be added to ensure the recipe is nutritionally complete.

Instructions: Cook the ground turkey: Ensure the ground turkey is thoroughly cooked, and set it aside to cool.

Prepare the sweet potatoes: Mash the sweet potatoes, providing a nutrient-rich carbohydrate source that complements the protein content of the turkey.

Combine ingredients: In a bowl, mix the cooked turkey, mashed sweet potatoes, chopped parsley, and a tablespoon of turkey or chicken broth

This results in a pleasing combination of tastes and textures.

Optional: Add taurine supplement: If not present in adequate amounts naturally, consult with your veterinarian to determine an appropriate taurine supplement and incorporate it into the mixture.

Serve the surprise: Portion the Turkey and Sweet Potato Surprise according to your cat's size and preferences. Observe your cat's reaction to ensure they enjoy and tolerate the homemade meal.

This recipe not only introduces variety into your cat's diet but also provides essential nutrients for their well-being. As with any homemade cat food, it's essential to consult with a veterinarian to ensure the recipe aligns with your cat's dietary requirements and health status.

Intermediate Recipes

Intermediate cat food recipes offer a step-up in complexity, providing more variety in flavors and nutrients for your feline companion. These recipes still maintain a focus on balanced nutrition while introducing a wider range of ingredients. Here are two intermediate recipes designed to elevate your cat's dining experience:

1. Tuna and Quinoa Medley:

Ingredients:

1/2 cup of canned tuna (in water, drained)

1/4 cup of cooked quinoa

1 tablespoon of finely chopped spinach

1 teaspoon of salmon oil (optional, for added omega-3 fatty acids)

1/4 teaspoon of taurine supplement (consult your veterinarian for appropriate dosage)

Instructions:

Combine the drained tuna, cooked quinoa, and finely chopped spinach in a mixing bowl.

To guarantee an equitable distribution of the components, carefully combine them.

Optional: Drizzle salmon oil over the mixture for an extra nutritional boost.

Add a taurine supplement, making sure it is well-mixed into the medley.

Portion and serve to your cat, adjusting quantities based on their size and dietary needs.

2. Salmon and Pumpkin Feast:

Ingredients:

1/2 cup of cooked and flaked salmon

1/4 cup of pureed pumpkin (unsweetened)

1 tablespoon of cooked green beans (finely chopped)

1 teaspoon of olive oil

1/4 teaspoon of taurine supplement (consult your veterinarian for appropriate dosage)

Instructions: Flake the cooked salmon into small, bite-sized pieces.

In a mixing bowl, combine the flaked salmon, pureed pumpkin, finely chopped green beans, and olive oil.

Mix the ingredients thoroughly, ensuring a well-blended consistency. Add a taurine supplement, ensuring it is evenly distributed in the feast.

Portion and serve to your cat, adjusting the serving size based on their individual needs.

These intermediate recipes introduce new protein sources, grains, and vegetables to diversify your cat's diet. As with any homemade cat food.

Tuna and Quinoa Medley

The "Tuna and Quinoa Medley" is an intermediate-level homemade cat food recipe that combines the savory flavors of tuna with the nutritional benefits of quinoa. This medley offers a well-rounded mix of proteins, essential amino acids, and wholesome grains for a cat's balanced nutrition. Here's a closer look at this delightful and nutritious recipe:

Ingredients: Canned tuna (in water, drained): Tuna provides a high-quality protein source that is not only delicious but also essential for muscle development and overall feline health.

Cooked quinoa: Quinoa is a nutrient-rich whole grain that adds complex carbohydrates, fiber, and various vitamins and minerals to the recipe.

Finely chopped spinach: Spinach contributes additional vitamins and minerals, enhancing the nutritional profile with a touch of green freshness.

Salmon oil (optional): Salmon oil introduces omega-3 fatty acids, promoting skin and coat health, and supporting overall well-being.

Taurine supplement (optional): Taurine is an essential amino acid for cats, and a supplement ensures that the recipe meets their specific dietary requirements.

Instructions: Combine the ingredients: In a mixing bowl, blend the drained tuna, cooked quinoa, and finely chopped spinach. Ensure the ingredients are evenly distributed for a balanced flavor profile.

Optional: Add salmon oil: Drizzle salmon oil over the mixture for an extra burst of flavor and the benefits of omega-3 fatty acids.

Adding the taurine supplement: If not present in sufficient amounts naturally, consult with your veterinarian to determine an appropriate taurine supplement dosage. Add it to the medley and mix well.

Serve to your cat: Portion the Tuna and Quinoa Medley according to your cat's size and dietary preferences. Observe their reaction to ensure they enjoy this nutritious and flavorful homemade meal.

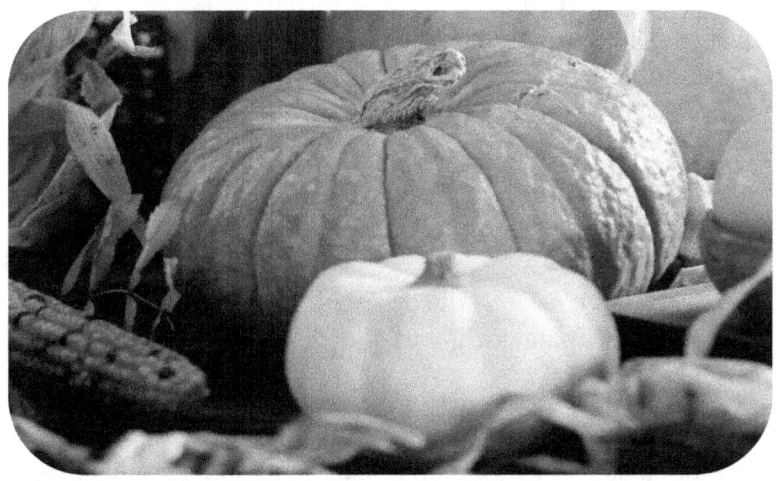

Salmon and Pumpkin Feast

The "Salmon and Pumpkin Feast" is an intermediate-level homemade cat food recipe that combines the rich flavors of salmon with the nutritional goodness of pumpkin. This feast offers a diverse range of nutrients, including omega-3 fatty acids, protein, and dietary fiber, making it a delightful and healthful option for your feline friend.

Ingredients: Cooked and flaked salmon: Salmon is a nutrient-dense fish that provides high-quality protein and essential omega-3 fatty acids, supporting heart health, joint function, and a glossy coat.

Pureed pumpkin (unsweetened): Pumpkin is a low-calorie, fiber-rich ingredient that aids in digestion, helps regulate bowel movements, and contributes to overall gastrointestinal health.

Cooked green beans (finely chopped): Green beans provide additional fiber and essential nutrients, adding a crunchy texture to the feast.

Olive oil: Olive oil introduces healthy monounsaturated fats, enhancing the palatability of the dish and promoting skin health.

Taurine supplement (optional): Taurine is a crucial amino acid for cats, and a supplement can be included to ensure the recipe meets their specific dietary requirements.

Instructions:

Flake the salmon: Thoroughly cook the salmon and flake it into small, bite-sized pieces, ensuring it is boneless and free from skin.

Prepare the pumpkin: Puree unsweetened pumpkin to add a rich, velvety texture to the feast. Pumpkin contributes dietary fiber and essential vitamins.

Combine the ingredients: In a mixing bowl, blend the flaked salmon, pureed pumpkin, finely chopped cooked green beans, and a teaspoon of olive oil. Mix the ingredients thoroughly to create a well-balanced and flavorful medley.

Optional: Add taurine supplement: If necessary, consult with your veterinarian to determine an appropriate taurine supplement dosage. Add it to the feast, ensuring it is evenly distributed.

Serve the feast: Portion the Salmon and Pumpkin Feast according to your cat's size and dietary preferences. Monitor their response to ensure they enjoy this nutritious and enticing homemade meal.

Advanced Recipe

Advanced cat food recipes take homemade feline nutrition to the next level, incorporating a wider array of ingredients to offer exceptional taste and diverse nutrients. These recipes cater to cat owners with confidence in preparing more complex meals. Here are two advanced recipes that go beyond the basics:

1. Gourmet Chicken and Shrimp Delicacy:

This exquisite dish combines lean chicken, succulent shrimp, and nutrient-rich vegetables. Ingredients may include boneless chicken thighs, fresh shrimp, steamed broccoli, and a splash of clam juice for added flavor. Precision in cooking methods and ingredient balance ensures a gourmet experience for your discerning feline.

2. Quail and Wild Rice Extravaganza:

This sophisticated recipe features quail, a lean poultry alternative, paired with the wholesome goodness of wild rice. Incorporating ingredients like asparagus, cranberries, and a dash of flaxseed oil, this dish provides a blend of flavors and textures, delivering a nutrient-rich feast for cats with refined tastes.

Beef and Liver Gourmet

The "Beef and Liver Gourmet" is an advanced cat food recipe designed to tantalize feline taste buds while delivering a robust nutritional profile. Combining the richness of beef with the nutrient-dense goodness of liver creates a gourmet experience for cats with discerning palates.

Ingredients:

Lean beef: A high-quality protein source that supports muscle development and overall feline health.

Liver: Packed with essential nutrients, including vitamins, minerals, and amino acids crucial for cats.

Sweet potatoes: Adding complex carbohydrates, fiber, and vitamins, sweet potatoes contribute to overall nutritional balance.

Blueberries: These antioxidant-rich berries enhance flavor while providing additional vitamins and minerals.

Flaxseed oil: A source of omega-3 fatty acids, promoting skin and coat health.

Instructions: Prepare the beef and liver: Cook the lean beef and liver thoroughly, ensuring it is finely minced or pureed for easy feline consumption.

Cook the sweet potatoes: Steam or boil sweet potatoes until they are soft and mashable.

Combine ingredients: In a mixing bowl, blend the cooked beef, liver, mashed sweet potatoes, blueberries, and a dash of flaxseed oil. Ensure a uniform mixture for a well-balanced meal.

Portion and serve: Serve the Beef and Liver Gourmet according to your cat's size and dietary needs. Observe your cat's enjoyment of this sophisticated culinary creation.

This advanced recipe not only satisfies a cat's taste preferences but also provides a diverse array of essential nutrients. Consultation with a veterinarian ensures that the Beef and Liver Gourmet aligns with your cat's specific dietary requirements, fostering optimal feline health and satisfaction.

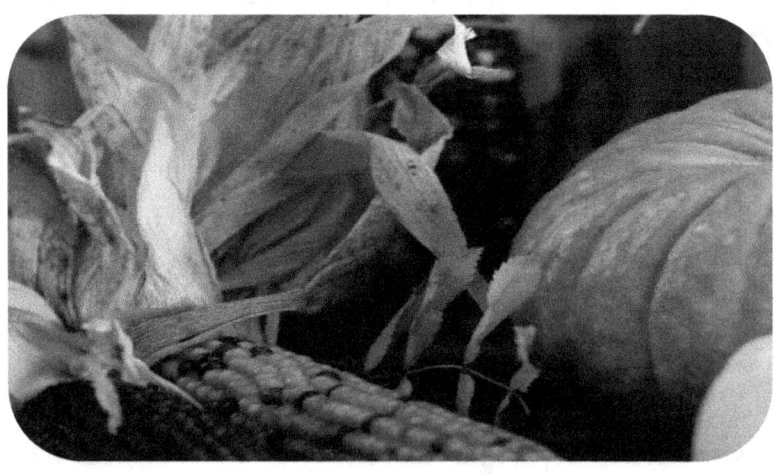

Homemade Fish and Vegetable Blend

The "Homemade Fish and Vegetable Blend" is an advanced cat food recipe that introduces a delightful fusion of aquatic flavors and nutrient-packed vegetables. This recipe not only appeals to cats with a penchant for seafood but also provides a comprehensive nutritional profile. Here's a glimpse into this sophisticated culinary creation:

Ingredients: Whitefish fillets: A lean source of protein that contributes to muscle development and overall feline health.

Salmon fillets: Rich in omega-3 fatty acids, supporting heart health and promoting a glossy coat.

Broccoli and carrots: These vegetables add vitamins, minerals, and dietary fiber, enhancing the overall nutritional balance of the blend.

Peas: Providing additional fiber and essential nutrients, peas contribute to digestive health.

Pumpkin puree: A nutrient-dense ingredient that aids in digestion, regulates bowel movements, and adds a velvety texture to the blend.

Instructions: Prepare the fish: Cook the whitefish and salmon fillets thoroughly, ensuring they are boneless and skinless, and flake them into bite-sized pieces.

Steam or boil vegetables: Cook the broccoli, carrots, and peas until they are tender, and finely chop them.

Combine ingredients: In a mixing bowl, blend the flaked fish, chopped vegetables, and pumpkin puree. Ensure an even distribution of ingredients for a harmonious flavor profile.

Portion and serve: Serve the Homemade Fish and Vegetable Blend according to your cat's size and dietary preferences. Observe their enjoyment of this advanced, nutritious, and delectable meal.

.

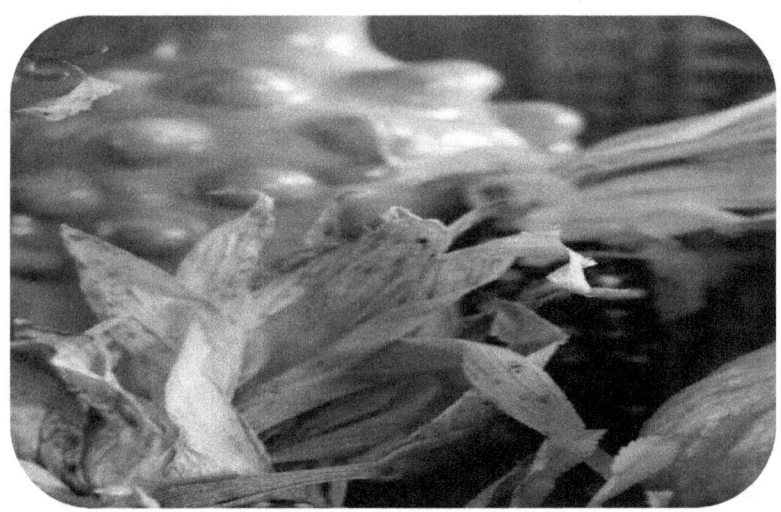

CHAPTER 5

SPECIAL DIETS AND HEALTH CONSIDERATIONS

Recipes for Cats with Allergies

Creating recipes for cats with allergies requires careful consideration and ingredient selection to address sensitivities and promote optimal health. Common allergens in cat food include certain proteins, grains, and additives. Here are guidelines for crafting hypoallergenic recipes:

1. Novel Protein Sources:

Choose novel protein sources that your cat hasn't been exposed to, such as rabbit, duck, or venison. These alternatives can be less likely to trigger allergic reactions.

2. Grain-Free Options:

Eliminate common grain allergens like wheat, corn, and soy. Opt for alternative carbohydrate sources such as sweet potatoes, peas, or lentils.

3. Limited Ingredients:

Keep recipes simple with a limited number of ingredients to minimize the chances of triggering allergies. This helps identify specific allergens more easily through an elimination diet.

4. Homemade Cat Food:

Prepare homemade cat food to have full control over the ingredients. This allows for customization based on your cat's specific allergens.

5. Allergen-Free Treats:

If offering treats, ensure they are also free from common allergens. Treats with a single protein source and minimal additives are preferable.

Example Recipe for Cats with Allergies:

Turkey and Pumpkin Delight:

Cooked ground turkey (novel protein)

Steamed and mashed pumpkin (digestive aid)

A small amount of olive oil (healthy fat)

Taurine supplement (essential amino acid for cats)

Combining novel proteins with easily digestible ingredients like pumpkin creates a hypoallergenic meal. However, it's crucial to consult with a veterinarian to identify specific allergens, formulate a suitable recipe, and ensure nutritional adequacy. Regular veterinary check-ups help monitor your cat's health and dietary adjustments as needed for their well-being.

Senior Cat Diet Plans

Senior cat diet plans are crucial for maintaining the health and well-being of older felines, addressing their changing nutritional needs as they age. Cats typically enter their senior years around the age of 7, and during this phase, adjustments to their diet can enhance their quality of life. Here are key considerations for creating a senior cat diet plan:

1. Lower Caloric Intake: Senior cats may have reduced activity levels, making them prone to weight gain. Adjusting their caloric intake helps prevent obesity and related health issues. However, it's essential to monitor weight changes and adjust portions accordingly.

2. Increased Protein Content: Aging cats may experience muscle loss, and maintaining a higher protein intake supports muscle mass. Opt for easily digestible protein sources, such as lean meats or high-quality commercial senior cat foods.

3. Joint and Mobility Support: Incorporate nutrients like omega-3 fatty acids and glucosamine to support joint health and mobility. These additions can alleviate stiffness and discomfort associated with aging joints.

4. Digestive Health: Senior cats may face digestive issues, so including easily digestible fibers from sources like pumpkin or rice can aid in digestion and prevent constipation.

5. Dental Care: Dental problems are common in older cats. Choose wet or soft foods to accommodate potential dental issues. Dental treats or adding water to dry kibble can also aid in oral health.

6. Regular Vet Check-ups: Consult with a veterinarian to determine the specific needs of your senior cat. Regular check-ups allow for adjustments to the diet based on any emerging health concerns or changing nutritional requirements.

7. Hydration: Older cats may be prone to dehydration, so ensure access to fresh water at all times. Wet food can contribute to overall hydration and is often more palatable for senior cats.

8. Limited Phosphorus for Renal Health: Kidney function may decline with age. Limiting phosphorus intake can be beneficial for senior cats, as it reduces the workload on the kidneys.

Example Senior Cat Diet Plan:

Ingredients: Cooked chicken or turkey (lean protein)

Cooked and mashed sweet potatoes (easily digestible carbohydrates)

Steamed green beans (fiber and nutrients)

Fish oil (omega-3 fatty acids for joint and skin health)

Taurine supplement (essential amino acid for cats)

Crafting a senior cat diet plan involves thoughtful consideration of these factors, ensuring that your cat's nutritional needs are met in their later years.

Homemade Food for Cats with Medical Conditions

Creating homemade food for cats with medical conditions requires careful consideration of the specific health issues your feline companion is facing. Whether its kidney disease, diabetes, allergies, or gastrointestinal problems, a tailored diet can play a crucial role in managing these conditions. Here are some general guidelines and considerations for preparing homemade cat food for various medical conditions:

1. Kidney Disease: Lower Phosphorus Content: Reduce phosphorus levels to ease the workload on the kidneys. Use lean meats such as chicken or turkey, and include egg whites instead of whole eggs.

Increased Omega-3 Fatty Acids: Incorporate fish oil or fatty fish like salmon for their omega-3 fatty acids, which can benefit cats with kidney disease.

2. Diabetes: High-Protein, Low-Carbohydrate: Opt for a diet high in protein to support muscle mass and low in carbohydrates to help regulate blood sugar levels. Use lean meats and include non-starchy vegetables like broccoli or spinach.

3. Gastrointestinal Issues: Easily Digestible Proteins: Choose easily digestible protein sources, such as boiled chicken or turkey, to minimize stress on the digestive system.

Plain Rice or Pumpkin: Incorporate plain rice or pumpkin, which can have a soothing effect on the digestive tract and aid in firming up stools.

4. Allergies: Novel Protein Sources: If your cat has food allergies, opt for novel protein sources like rabbit or duck. Exclude common allergens such as beef, chicken, or grains.

5. Hyperthyroidism: Balanced Iodine Content: Be cautious with iodine-rich ingredients like fish, as excessive iodine can exacerbate hyperthyroidism. Consult with a veterinarian to determine suitable iodine levels in the diet.

6. Weight Management:

Calorie Control: For cats needing weight management, carefully control calorie intake. Use lean proteins, limit fats, and include high-fiber vegetables to create a satisfying meal without excess calories.

7. Inflammatory Bowel Disease (IBD):

Hypoallergenic Proteins: Choose hypoallergenic proteins like venison or rabbit. Steam or cook vegetables to make them easier to digest.

Recipe for Cats with Kidney Disease:

Ingredients:

Cooked chicken or turkey (lean protein)

Egg whites (low phosphorus protein source)

Fish oil (omega-3 fatty acids)

White rice (limited phosphorus)

Steamed green beans (fiber)

Taurine supplement (essential amino acid for cats)

CHAPTER 6

Tips for Feeding Homemade Cat Food

Transitioning Your Cat to Homemade Food

Transitioning your cat to homemade food requires a gradual and patient approach to ensure a smooth adjustment to the new diet. Cats can be particularly sensitive to changes in their food, so a thoughtful transition plan is essential for their well-being.

1. Consult with a Veterinarian: Before starting the transition, consult with your veterinarian to determine the appropriate nutritional requirements for your cat. The veterinarian can provide guidance on the specific needs of your cat, taking into account factors such as age, weight, and any existing health conditions.

2. Choose a Balanced Recipe: Select a balanced homemade cat food recipe that meets the nutritional needs of your feline companion. Ensure it includes a proper balance of proteins, fats, carbohydrates, vitamins, and minerals.

3. Gradual Transition: Start the transition by mixing a small amount of homemade food with your cat's current commercial diet. Gradually increase the proportion of homemade food while decreasing the commercial food over the course of 7-10 days.

4. Monitor Behavior and Health: Observe your cat's behavior, energy levels, and overall health throughout the transition. Any signs of digestive upset, such as vomiting or diarrhea, should be addressed promptly. If issues persist, consult your veterinarian for guidance.

5. Ensure Hydration: Homemade cat food may have a higher water content, but it's still essential to ensure your cat stays adequately hydrated. Provide fresh water at all times to support their overall health.

6. Be Patient and Flexible: Cats can be creatures of habit, and they may initially resist changes to their diet. During the changeover period, be patient and understanding. If your cat is particularly resistant, consider introducing new flavors gradually or trying different protein sources.

7. Rotate Ingredients: Once your cat has successfully transitioned to homemade food, consider rotating protein sources and ingredients to provide variety and a broader range of nutrients. This can help prevent dietary deficiencies and keep mealtime interesting for your cat.

8. Regular Veterinary Check-ups: Schedule regular check-ups with your veterinarian to monitor your cat's health and nutritional status. This allows for adjustments to the homemade diet as needed and ensures your cat's well-being over time.

Transitioning your cat to homemade food requires careful planning, patience, and a vigilant eye on their overall health. By following a gradual transition plan, monitoring your cat's response, and working closely with your veterinarian, you can provide a balanced and nutritious homemade diet that supports your cat's unique needs and preferences.

Monitoring Your Cat's Health

Monitoring your cat's health is a crucial aspect of responsible pet ownership, ensuring their well-being and detecting potential issues early on. Regular monitoring involves a combination of observation, regular veterinary check-ups, and awareness of changes in behavior or physical condition.

1. Regular Veterinary Check-ups: Schedule routine veterinary appointments, ideally at least once a year, for thorough health assessments. These check-ups include examinations, vaccinations, and discussions about your cat's diet, behavior, and any changes in their routine.

2. Observation of Behavior: Pay close attention to your cat's behavior, noting any changes in activity levels, appetite, grooming habits, or litter box behavior. Behavioral changes can be indicative of underlying health issues.

3. Weight Management: Check your cat's weight on a regular basis to ensure it is within a healthy range. Sudden weight loss or gain can be a sign of various health problems, including metabolic issues or digestive disorders.

4. Dental Health: Check your cat's teeth and gums regularly for signs of dental issues, such as tartar buildup, redness, or swelling. Dental problems can lead to other health issues if left unaddressed.

5. Coat and Skin Condition: A cat's coat is a reflection of their overall health. A shiny, clean coat suggests good nutrition, while changes in fur texture, excessive shedding, or skin abnormalities may indicate underlying health concerns.

6. Litter Box Monitoring: Keep a watch on your cat's toilet habits. Changes in urine or feces, including frequency, consistency, or the presence of blood, can signal health issues such as urinary tract infections or gastrointestinal problems.

7. Eating Habits: Monitor your cat's eating habits, noting any changes in appetite or preferences. Sudden changes in eating behavior can be indicative of dental problems, digestive issues, or underlying health conditions.

8. Respiratory Health: Observe your cat's breathing patterns. Labored breathing, coughing, or sneezing may be signs of respiratory issues that require veterinary attention.

9. Eye and Ear Health: Regularly check your cat's eyes and ears for signs of redness, discharge, or unusual odors. These could be indicative of infections or other issues.

10. Age-Related Monitoring: Be aware of age-related changes in your cat's health, such as arthritis, reduced mobility, or changes in activity levels. Senior cats may require more frequent veterinary check-ups and specialized care.

By actively monitoring your cat's health through regular veterinary visits and attentive observation, you can catch potential issues early and provide timely intervention. Establishing a strong partnership with your veterinarian ensures comprehensive care and promotes a long, healthy life for your feline companion.

Troubleshooting Common Issues

Troubleshooting common issues in cats involves identifying and addressing problems that may affect their health, behavior, or overall well-being. While some issues may be minor and easily resolved, others may require veterinary attention. Here are common problems and troubleshooting tips for cat owners:

**1. Digestive Upset:

Symptoms: Vomiting, diarrhea, or constipation.

Troubleshooting: Identify recent changes in diet, eliminate potential toxic substances, and ensure access to fresh water. If issues persist, consult a veterinarian.

**2. Urinary Issues:

Symptoms: Straining to urinate, frequent urination, blood in urine.

Troubleshooting: Ensure access to a clean litter box, monitor water intake, and provide a balanced diet. If symptoms persist, seek veterinary advice to rule out urinary tract infections or other issues.

**3. Behavioral Changes:

Symptoms: Aggression, excessive grooming, changes in litter box habits.

Troubleshooting: Evaluate environmental stressors, changes in routine, or the introduction of new pets. If behavioral issues persist, consult with a veterinarian or a feline behavior specialist.

**4. Weight Management:

Symptoms: Sudden weight loss or gain.

Troubleshooting: Adjust portion sizes, monitor feeding habits, and consider a balanced, portion-controlled diet. If weight issues persist, consult a veterinarian to rule out underlying health conditions.

**5. Dental Problems:

Symptoms: Bad breath, reluctance to eat, pawing at the mouth.

Troubleshooting: Introduce dental care routines, such as tooth brushing or dental treats. Regular veterinary check-ups can address dental issues and prevent further complications.

**6. Allergies:

Symptoms: Itchy skin, redness, gastrointestinal upset.

Troubleshooting: Identify potential allergens in the diet, such as certain proteins or additives. Transition to a hypoallergenic diet and consult with a veterinarian for further guidance.

**7. Hairballs:

Symptoms: Frequent coughing, hacking, or vomiting of hairballs.

Troubleshooting: Regular grooming to reduce shedding, introducing hairball remedies or special diets, and ensuring access to fresh water can help manage hairball issues.

8. Respiratory Issues:

Symptoms: Sneezing, coughing, nasal discharge.

Troubleshooting: Ensure a clean environment, monitor for signs of respiratory infections, and seek veterinary attention if symptoms persist.

9. Joint Problems:

Symptoms: Reduced mobility, stiffness, or reluctance to jump.

Troubleshooting: Provide a comfortable environment, consider joint supplements, and consult with a veterinarian for tailored management, especially in senior cats.

10. Anxiety or Stress:

Symptoms: Excessive grooming, hiding, changes in appetite.

Troubleshooting: Identify stressors and provide a calm environment. Consider pheromone diffusers or calming products. Seek professional advice if needed.

Troubleshooting common issues in cats requires a combination of observation, preventive care, and prompt veterinary intervention when necessary. Regular veterinary check-ups and open communication with your veterinarian play a crucial role in maintaining your cat's health and addressing issues early on.

CHAPTER 7

FREQUENTLY ASKED QUESTIONS

How Much Homemade Food Should I Feed My Cat?

Determining the appropriate amount of homemade food to feed your cat requires careful consideration of several factors, including your cat's weight, age, activity level, and any underlying health conditions. Unlike commercial cat foods with feeding guidelines on the packaging, homemade diets need to be tailored to meet your cat's specific nutritional needs. Here's a general guide to help you determine the right amount of homemade food for your feline friend:

1. Calculate Caloric Needs: Start by calculating your cat's daily caloric needs. Factors such as age, weight, activity level, and health status influence calorie requirements. Your veterinarian can help you determine an appropriate daily caloric intake for your cat.

2. Protein Requirements: Cats are obligate carnivores, and their diets should be rich in high-quality protein. Ensure that the homemade food provides an adequate amount of protein, usually around 25-40% of the total caloric intake.

3. Monitor Weight and Body Condition:

Regularly monitor your cat's weight and body condition. Adjust the portion size based on whether your cat needs to gain or lose weight. Veterinarians use body condition scoring to assess if a cat is underweight, overweight, or at an ideal weight.

4. Consider Macronutrient Balance: Aim for a balanced diet that includes an appropriate mix of proteins, fats, and carbohydrates. While cats don't require carbohydrates in large amounts, they can contribute to overall nutritional balance.

5. Feed in Multiple Small Meals: Cats are natural grazers, and feeding them small, frequent meals throughout the day mimics their natural eating behavior. This approach also helps prevent overeating and supports digestion.

6. Adjust Based on Health Conditions: If your cat has specific health conditions, such as kidney disease or diabetes, work closely with your veterinarian to adjust the homemade diet accordingly. Certain medical conditions may require specific dietary modifications.

7. Consult with a Veterinarian: Regular veterinary check-ups are crucial for monitoring your cat's health and adjusting their diet as needed. Consult with your veterinarian to ensure the homemade diet meets your cat's nutritional requirements.

8. Monitor Hydration: Homemade diets may have a different moisture content compared to commercial cat food. Monitor your cat's water intake to ensure they remain adequately hydrated.

As a starting point, a typical adult cat may require around 200-300 calories per day, but individual needs can vary widely. It's essential to be flexible and make adjustments based on your cat's specific requirements. Always consult with your veterinarian for personalized guidance on portion sizes and dietary compositions.

Can I Use Raw Ingredients in Cat Food?

You can use raw ingredients in cat food, and many cat owners opt for a raw or partially raw diet to mimic a more natural and species-appropriate feeding approach. However, using raw ingredients requires careful handling and consideration to ensure the safety and nutritional completeness of the diet.

When incorporating raw ingredients into your cat's food:

Quality Matters: Choose high-quality, fresh, and, if possible, organic ingredients. This includes selecting fresh meats, organs, and other components that are fit for human consumption.

Nutritional Balance: Ensure the diet is nutritionally balanced, providing the necessary proteins, fats, vitamins, and minerals essential for a cat's health. This may involve incorporating a variety of meats, organs, and supplements.

Hygiene and Safety: Practice excellent hygiene to prevent contamination and reduce the risk of foodborne illnesses. Thoroughly wash hands, utensils, and surfaces when handling raw ingredients.

Supplements: Depending on the ingredients used, you may need to add supplements like taurine, which is crucial for cats and can degrade during the cooking process.

Transition Gradually: If transitioning from commercial cat food to a raw diet, do so gradually. Cats can be sensitive to dietary changes, and a slow transition helps prevent digestive upset.

Consult with a Veterinarian: Before starting a raw diet, consult with your veterinarian. They can provide guidance on the nutritional requirements, potential supplements, and help tailor a raw feeding plan that suits your cat's individual needs.

While raw diets can offer benefits such as improved coat condition and dental health, it's essential to be well-informed, maintain strict hygiene practices, and work closely with your veterinarian to ensure your cat's nutritional needs are met and their health is safeguarded. Regular veterinary check-ups help monitor your cat's overall health and allow for adjustments to their diet as needed.

What Supplements are Necessary for Homemade Cat Food?

When preparing homemade cat food, it's crucial to ensure that the diet is nutritionally complete and balanced. While whole foods contribute to many essential nutrients, some supplements may be necessary to meet specific dietary requirements for cats. Here are key supplements often recommended for homemade cat food:

Taurine: Taurine is an essential amino acid for cats, critical for heart health and vision. It's commonly found in meat, but cooking can reduce its content. Taurine supplementation is often necessary to ensure sufficient levels.

Vitamins and Minerals: Commercial cat foods are fortified with essential vitamins and minerals. In homemade diets, it's important to provide a broad spectrum of these nutrients. A feline multivitamin or individual supplements for specific vitamins (like vitamin D or B-complex) may be needed.

Calcium: Adequate calcium is crucial for bone health. If the homemade diet lacks sufficient bone content, calcium supplements such as calcium carbonate may be necessary. However, getting the balance right is vital to prevent deficiencies or excess.

Fish Oil or Omega-3 Fatty Acids: Fish oil is a source of omega-3 fatty acids, which support skin and coat health, reduce inflammation, and provide cardiovascular benefits. Including fish oil or other omega-3 supplements ensures these essential fatty acids are present.

Fiber: Some homemade diets may lack sufficient fiber. Adding psyllium husk or other fiber supplements can help regulate digestion and prevent constipation.

Probiotics: Probiotics improve intestinal health by encouraging the development of healthy microorganisms. They can be especially helpful for cats with digestive issues or those transitioning to a new diet.

Iodine: If your cat's diet lacks sufficient iodine, often found in fish or iodized salt, iodine supplements may be necessary to support thyroid function.

Lysine: Lysine is a necessary amino acid that aids in immunological function. Cats may need additional lysine supplementation, especially during periods of stress or illness.

Before adding any supplements to your cat's diet, contact with a veterinarian. Each cat is unique, and their nutritional requirements may differ. A veterinarian can assess your cat's health, advice on necessary supplements, and ensure that the homemade diet meets their specific requirements. Regular veterinary check-ups are essential for monitoring your cat's overall health and making any necessary adjustments to their diet over time.

Appendix: Resources and References

Recommended Reading

"Dr. Becker's Real Food for Healthy Dogs and Cats" by Karen Becker and Beth Taylor is a recommended resource for in-depth insights about homemade cat food.

The book offers practical guidance on creating nutritionally balanced meals for pets. Donald R. Strombeck's "Home-Prepared Dog and Cat Diets: The Healthful Alternative" is another great resource, giving thorough information on constructing homemade diets to fulfill a pet's nutritional needs. Always consult with a veterinarian for personalized advice, and these resources can complement your understanding of crafting wholesome meals for your feline friend.

Online Resources for Cat Nutrition

Explore reputable online resources like the American Association of Feed Control Officials (AAFCO) website for guidelines on pet food regulations. The World Small Animal Veterinary Association (WSAVA) provides valuable information on pet nutrition. Websites such as PetMD and the Cornell Feline Health Center offer articles and guides on cat nutrition. Additionally, platforms like Balance IT and the National Research Council's Nutrient Requirements of Dogs and Cats can assist in formulating balanced homemade cat diets. Always cross-reference information and consult with a veterinarian to ensure the advice aligns with your cat's specific health needs.

CONCLUSION

As we turn the final page of this cookbook, it's not merely a conclusion but a celebration of the remarkable bond you share with your beloved feline friends. This culinary guide has been more than a collection of recipes; it's been an exploration into the heart of your kitchen, where love and nutrition harmonize to create meals that transcend the ordinary.

Within these pages, we've delved into the art of crafting homemade cat food – from understanding the nuanced nutritional needs of our whiskered companions to embracing the joy of cooking with love. Each recipe is a testament to the care you invest in your cat's well-being, transforming mealtime into a moment of connection and delight.

The decision to prepare your cat's meals at home is a commitment to their health and happiness. It's an acknowledgment that our feline friends are not just pets but cherished members of the family, deserving of the best we can offer. This cookbook is not merely a guide; it's an invitation to embark on an extraordinary journey of providing wholesome, homemade goodness to those who enrich our lives with their presence.

As you close this chapter, take with you the satisfaction of knowing that every ingredient, every measured portion, and every aromatic creation was a gesture of love. The kitchen has become a place where the culinary and the sentimental intertwine, where a simple act of preparing a meal becomes an expression of devotion.

Remember, our whiskered friends are not just recipients of our care; they are silent companions through life's journey. The joyous purrs, the playful antics, and the comforting presence on lazy afternoons – these are the threads that weave the tapestry of a life shared with a cat. And in the midst of this tapestry, the meals you prepare are the vibrant colors that add richness and depth to the experience.

While this cookbook serves as a comprehensive guide, it's also an invitation to continue exploring, learning, and innovating in the kitchen. Feel free to experiment with flavors, ingredients, and even presentation. After all, the joy of cooking for your cat lies not just in the result but in the process, the shared moments, and the endless possibilities.

In the spirit of this culinary adventure, take a moment to reflect on the journey you've undertaken. From the first cautious attempt at preparing a homemade meal to the confident mastery of crafting a balanced, nutritious feast – it's a testament to your dedication and love. Your cat may not express gratitude in words, but in the twinkle of their eyes and the contentment of their purrs, you'll find the most sincere appreciation.

As you bid adieu, let this be a Launchpad for continued exploration and a source of inspiration for countless future meals. Share your culinary discoveries with fellow cat enthusiasts, and let the joy of homemade cat food ripple through our feline-loving community. Thank you for allowing this guide to be a part of your kitchen, your home, and your heart. May your cat's bowl always be filled with the warmth of homemade goodness, and may every mealtime be a celebration of the extraordinary bond you share. Happy cooking, happy whiskers, and happy trails on this beautiful journey with your feline companions.

www.ingramcontent.com/pod-product-compliance
Lightning Source LLC
Chambersburg PA
CBHW070117010626
45794CB00013B/2563